The Ultimate Lean And Green Cookbook For Beginners

Proven Strategies On A Complete Lean And Green Diet Book With Effortless Lean And Green Recipes To Lose Weight By Harnessing The Power Of "Fuelings Hacks Meal

Natalie Allen

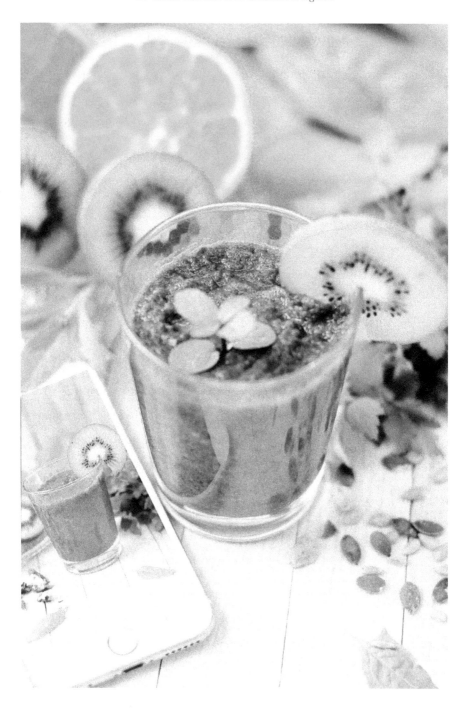

TABLE OF CONTENTS

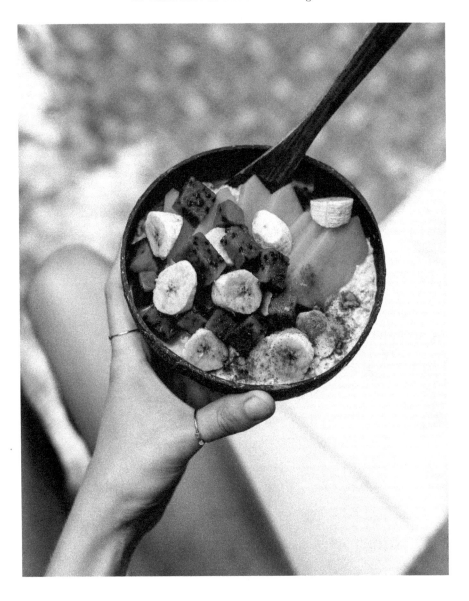

Introduction

One way is by changing your diet and cooking in a smarter way. Lean and Green Cookbook provides recipes for delicious, healthy food with reduced environmental impact. Get ready to cook up a storm that's good for the environment!

This article was written because there are so many people who want tips and tricks on how to stay lean while reducing their environmental impact. It does not matter if you are a novice or a pro chef; this book will educate and inspire a way to make the best out of the foods you eat. Eat healthy with dietary guidelines in mind. s

The cookbook is full of a little bit of everything from main dishes to light breakfasts. From protein-packed animal and seafood recipes to balanced and delicious vegetarian and vegan dishes. So, get ready for a feast on the go! You'll be amazed just how tasty healthy can be in a nutshell.

Lean and Green is perfect for people who want to cook healthy food without a lot of hassle or spending a lot of time in the kitchen. It includes easy recipes that take 30 minutes or less to make, making it ideal for busy people with hectic schedules. In addition, the book is also loaded with nutritional information about every recipe, including calories, fat, carbohydrates, and protein content.

Vegetarian Delicacies: Everything you need to know about vegetarian cuisine. These dishes include Mexican, Italian, Chinese, Indian, Thai, Greek, French, Japanese, and Taiwanese. The recipes are based on traditional food from these countries that are healthy without being bland or boring. These recipes are also vegan and gluten-free.

Everything you need to know about vegetarian cuisine. These dishes include Mexican, Italian, Chinese, Indian, Thai, Greek, French, Japanese and Taiwanese. The recipes are based on traditional food from these countries that are healthy without being bland or boring. These recipes are also vegan and gluten-free. Heartiest Dishes: These dishes are full of protein and carbohydrates as well as vitamins and minerals. The meals are hearty but leave you feeling full so you don't need to eat constantly. They feature a variety of meats, beans and vegetables. These dishes make great entrees or side dishes.

These dishes are full of protein and carbohydrates as well as vitamins and minerals. The meals are hearty but leave you feeling full so you don't need to eat constantly. They feature a variety of meats, beans and vegetables. These dishes make great entrees or side dishes. Energy Boosts: These dishes are tasty and nutritious but also relatively low in calories. They will provide the boost you need to recover from a hard workout or day at work.

Most people don't have time to cook healthy food, but that doesn't mean it's out of the question. On the contrary, people should always be trying to incorporate healthy eating into their lives. There are many ways for you to do this, such as making changes to your diet or stocking your pantry with nutritious ingredients. This will help you better control your diabetes and overall health.

21 Days Meal Plan

Day	Breakfast	Lunch	Dinner	Dessert
1	Basil Tomato Frittata	Almond Pancakes	Zucchini Salmon Salad	Spinach and Artichoke Dip
2	Coconut Bread	Mouth-watering Pie	Pan Fried Salmon	Buffalo Dip
3	Chia Spinach Pancakes	Peanut Butter and Cacao Breakfast Quinoa	Grilled Salmon with Pineapple Salsa	Potato Wedges
4	Olive Cheese Omelet	Chicken Omelet	Mediterranean Chickpea Salad	Dill Hummus
5	Feta Kale Frittata	Almond Coconut Cereal	Warm Chorizo Chickpea Salad	Latte Pudding
6	Fresh Berry Muffins	WW Salad in a Jar	Tomato Fish Bake	Peanut Butter
7	Cheese Zucchini Eggplant	Almond Porridge	Garlicky Tomato Chicken Casserole	Vegan Crackers
8	Broccoli Nuggets	Special Almond Cereal	Chicken Cacciatore	Spelt Banana Bread
9	Cauliflower Frittata	Bacon and Lemon spiced Muffins	Fennel Wild Rice Risotto	Yeast-Free Spelt Bread
10	Coconut Kale Muffins	Greek Style Mini Burger Pies	Wild Rice Prawn Salad	Flatbread

11	Protein Muffins	Awesome Avocado Muffins	Chicken Broccoli Salad with Avocado Dressing	Chickpea Loaf
12	Healthy Waffles	Raw-Cinnamon-Apple Nut Bowl	Seafood Paella	Zucchini Bread Pancakes
13	Cheese Almond Pancakes	Family Fun Pizza	Herbed Roasted Chicken Breasts	Kamut and Raisin Pancakes
14	Vegetable Quiche	Tasty WW Pancakes	Marinated Chicken Breasts	Spelt and Strawberry Waffles
15	Pumpkin Muffins	Slow Cooker Savory Butternut Squash Oatmeal	Greek Style Quesadillas	Chickpea and Quinoa Burgers
16	Pancakes with Berries	Yummy Smoked Salmon	Creamy Penne	Teff Burgers
17	Omelette À La Margherita	WW Breakfast Cereal	Light Paprika Moussaka	Chickpea Nuggets
18	Porridge with Walnuts	Avocados Stuffed with Salmon	Cucumber Bowl with Spices and Greek Yogurt	Pumpkin Spice Crackers
19	Alkaline Blueberry Spelt Pancakes	Green Lamb Curry	Stuffed Bell Peppers with Quinoa	Spicy Roasted Nuts
20	Ancho Tilapia on Cauliflower Rice	Lemon Lamb Chops	Mediterranean Burrito	Potato Chips

Breakfast Recipes

1. Hash BrownPreparation Time: 15 Minutes

Cooking Time: 15 Minutes

Servings: 4

Ingredients:

- 1 pound russet potatoes, peeled, processed using a grater

- Pinch of sea salt

- Pinch of black pepper, to taste

- 3 Tbsp. Olive oil

Directions:

1.   Line a microwave safe-dish with paper towels. Spread shredded

potatoes on top—microwave veggies on the highest heat setting for 2

minutes. Remove from heat.

2.   Pour one tablespoon of oil into a non-stick skillet set over medium heat.

3.   Cooking in batches, place a generous pinch of potatoes into the hot oil. Press down using the back of a spatula.

4.   Cook for 3 minutes on every side, or until brown and crispy. Drain on paper towels—repeat the step for the remaining potatoes. Add more oil as needed.

5.   Season with salt and pepper. Serve.

Nutrition:

Calories: 200 kcal

Protein: 4.03g

Fat: 11.73g

Carbohydrates: 20.49g

2. Apple Ginger and Rhubarb Muffins

Preparation Time: 15 Minutes

Cooking Time: 25 Minutes

Servings: 4

Ingredients:

- ½ Cup Finely ground almonds

- ¼ Cup Brown rice flour

- ½ Cup Buckwheat flour

- 1/8 Cup Unrefined raw sugar

- 2 Tbsp. Arrowroot flour

- 1 Tbsp. Linseed meal

- 2 Tbsp. Crystallized ginger, finely chopped

- ½ Tsp. Ground ginger

- ½ Tsp. Ground cinnamon

- 2 Tsp. Gluten-free baking powder

- A pinch of fine sea salt

- 1 small apple, peeled and finely diced

- 1 cup finely chopped rhubarb

- 1/3 cup almond/ rice milk

- 1 Large egg

- ¼ cup extra virgin olive oil

- 1 Tsp. Pure vanilla extract

Directions:

1. Set your oven to 350°F grease an eight-cup muffin tin and line with paper cases.

2. Combine the almond four, linseed meal, ginger, salt, and sugar in a mixing bowl. Sieve this mixture over the other flours, spices, and baking powder and use a whisk to combine well.

3. Stir in the apple and rhubarb in the flour mixture until evenly coated.

4.   In a separate bowl, whisk the milk, vanilla, and egg, then pour it into the dry mixture. Stir until just combined—don't overwork the batter as this can yield very tough muffins.

5.   Grease a muffin pan with oil. Scoop the mixture and top with a few slices of rhubarb. Bake for at least 25 minutes till they start turning golden or when an inserted toothpick emerges clean.

6.   Take off from the oven and let sit for at least 5 minutes before transferring the muffins to a wire rack for further cooling.

7.   Serve warm with a glass of squeezed juice.

8.   Enjoy!

Nutrition:

Calories: 325 kcal

Protein: 6.32g

Fat: 9.82g

Carbohydrates: 55.71g

3. Anti-Inflammatory Breakfast Frittata

Preparation Time: 10 Minutes

Cooking Time: 40 Minutes

Servings: 4

Ingredients:

- 4 large eggs

- 6 Egg whites

- 450g Button mushrooms

- 450g Baby spinach

- 125g Firm tofu

- 1 Onion, chopped

- 1 Tbsp. Minced garlic

- ½ Tsp. Ground turmeric

- ½ Tsp. Cracked black pepper

- ¼ Cup water

- Kosher salt to taste

Directions:

1. Set your oven to 350°F.

2. Sauté the mushrooms in a little bit of extra virgin olive oil in a large non-stick ovenproof pan over medium heat. Add the onions once the mushrooms start turning golden and cook for 3 minutes until the onions become soft.

3. Stir in the garlic, then cook for at least 30 seconds until fragrant before adding the spinach. Pour in water, cover, and cook until the spinach becomes wilted for about 2 minutes.

4. Take off the lid and continue cooking up until the water evaporates. Now, combine the eggs, egg whites, tofu, pepper, turmeric, and salt in a bowl. When all the liquid has evaporated, pour in the egg mixture, let cook for about 2 minutes until the edges start setting, then transfer to the oven and bake for about 25 minutes or until cooked.

5. Take off from the oven, then let sit for at least 5 minutes before cutting it into quarters and serving.

6.   Enjoy!

•   Tip: Baby spinach and mushrooms boost the nutrient profile of

the eggs to provide you with amazing anti-inflammatory benefits.

Nutrition:

Calories: 521 kcal

Protein: 29.13g

Fat: 10.45g

Carbohydrates: 94.94g

Lunch Recipes

4. Chicken Omelet

Preparation Time: 5 minutes

Cooking Time: 15 minutes

Servings: 1

Ingredients:

- 2 bacon slices; cooked and crumbled

- 2 eggs

- 1 tablespoon of homemade mayonnaise

- 1 tomato; chopped.

- 1-ounce of rotisserie chicken; shredded

- 1 teaspoon of mustard

- 1 small avocado; pitted, peeled and chopped.

- Salt and black pepper to the taste.

Directions:

1. In a bowl, mix eggs with some salt and pepper and whisk gently.

2. Heat up a pan over medium heat, spray with some vegetable oil, add eggs and cook your omelet for 5 minutes. Add chicken, avocado, tomato, bacon, mayo and mustard on one half of the omelet.

3. Fold omelet, cover pan and cook for 5 minutes more.

4. Transfer to a plate and serve.

Nutrition:

Calories: 400

Fat: 32 g

Fiber: 6 g

Carbs: 4 g

Protein: 25 g

5. Almond Coconut Cereal

Preparation Time: 5 minutes

Cooking Time: 5 minutes

Servings: 2

Ingredients:

- 1/3 cup of Water.

- 1/3 cup of Coconut milk.

- 2 tbsps. of Roasted sunflower seeds.

- 1 tbsp. of Chia seeds.

- ½ cup of Blueberries.

- 2 tbsps. of Chopped almonds.

Directions:

1. Put a medium bowl in position and add coconut milk and chia seeds, then put aside for 5 minutes.

2. Blend almond with sunflower seeds, then add the mixture to the chia seeds mixture and add water to make them mix evenly.

3. Serve topped with the remaining sunflower seeds and blueberries.

Nutrition:

Calories: 181

Fat: 15.2 g

Fiber: 4 g

Carbs: 10.8 g

Protein: 3.7 g

6. WW Salad in a Jar

Preparation Time: 10 minutes Cooking Time: 5 minutes

Servings: 1

Ingredients:

- 1-ounce of favorite greens

- 1-ounce of red bell pepper; chopped.

- 4 ounces of rotisserie chicken; roughly chopped.

- 4 tablespoons of extra virgin olive oil

- 1/2 scallion; chopped.

- 1-ounce of cucumber; chopped.

- 1-ounce of cherry tomatoes; halved

- Salt and black pepper to taste.

Directions:

1. In a bowl, mix greens with red bell pepper, tomatoes, scallion,

   cucumber, salt, pepper, olive oil, and toss to coat well.

2. Transfer this to a jar, top with chicken pieces and serve for breakfast.

Nutrition:

Calories: 180

Fat: 12 g

Fiber: 4 g

Carbs: 5 g

Protein: 17 g

Dinner Recipes

7. Cauliflower Rice

Preparation: 5 minutes Cooking: 20 minutes Servings: 1

Ingredients:

Round 1:

1.   1/2 tsp. turmeric 2.   1/2 cup of diced carrot

3.   1/8 cup of diced onion 4.   1/2 tbsp. low-sodium soy sauce

5.   1/8 block of extra firm tofu

Round 2:

*   1/2 cup of frozen peas

*   1/4 minced garlic cloves

*   1/2 cup of chopped broccoli

*   1/2 tbsp. minced ginger

*   1/4 tbsp. rice vinegar

- 1/4 tsp. toasted sesame oil

- 1/2 tbsp. reduced-sodium soy sauce

- 1/2 cup of riced cauliflower

Directions:

1. Crush tofu in a large bowl and toss with all the Round one ingredient.

2. Lock the air fryer lid — preheat the Instant Crisp Air Fryer to 370 degrees. Also, set the temperature to 370°F, set time to 10 minutes, and cook 10 minutes, making sure to shake once.

3. In another bowl, toss ingredients from Round 2 together.

4. Add Round 2 mixture to Instant Crisp Air Fryer and cook another 10 minutes to shake 5 minutes.

5. Enjoy!

Nutrition: Calories: 67 Fat: 8 g Protein: 3 g

Sugar: 0 g

8. Zucchini Omelet

Preparation Time: 10 minutes

Cooking Time: 10 minutes

Servings: 1

Ingredients:

- 1/2 teaspoon butter

- 1/2 zucchini, julienned

- One egg

- 1/8 teaspoon fresh basil, chopped

- 1/8 teaspoon red pepper flakes, crushed

- Salted and newly ground black pepper, to taste

Directions:

1.   Preheat the Instant Crisp Air Fryer to 355 degrees F.

2.   Melt butter on a medium heat using a skillet.

3.   Add zucchini and cook for about 3-4 minutes.

4.   In a bowl, add the eggs, basil, red pepper flakes, salt, and black pepper and beat well.

5.   Add cooked zucchini and gently stir to combine.

6.   Transfer the mixture into the Instant Crisp Air Fryer pan. Lock the air fryer lid.

7.   Cook for about 10 minutes. Also, you may opt to wait until it is done thoroughly.

Nutrition:

Calories: 285

Fat: 20.5 g

Protein: 8.6 g

9. Cheesy Cauliflower Fritters

Preparation Time: 10 minutes

Cooking Time: 7 minutes

Servings: 1

Ingredients:

- 1/2 cup of chopped parsley

- 1 cup of Italian breadcrumbs

- 1/3 cup of shredded mozzarella cheese

- 1/3 cup of shredded sharp cheddar cheese

- One egg

- Two minced garlic cloves

- Three chopped scallions

- One head of cauliflower

Directions:

1.   Cut the cauliflower up into florets. Wash well and pat dry. Place

into a food processor and pulse 20-30 seconds till it looks like rice.

2.	Place the cauliflower rice in a bowl and mix with pepper, salt, egg, cheeses, breadcrumbs, garlic, and scallions.

3.	With hands, form 15 patties of the mixture, and then add more breadcrumbs if needed.

4.	With olive oil, spritz patties, and put the fitters into your Instant Crisp Air Fryer. Pile it in a single layer. Lock the air fryer lid. Set temperature to 390°F, and set time to 7 minutes, flipping after 7 minutes.

Nutrition:

Calories: 209

Fat: 17 g

Protein: 6 g

Sugar: 0.5 g

Meat Recipes

10. Beef Stroganoff

Preparation Time: 10 Minutes

Cooking Time: 14 Minutes

Servings: 4

Ingredients:

• 9 Oz. Tender Beef

• 1 Onion, chopped

• 1 Tbsp. Paprika

• 3/4 Cup Sour Cream

• Salt and Pepper to taste

• Baking Dish

Directions:

1. Preheat the Cuisinart Air Fryer Oven to 390 degrees.

2. Chop the beef and marinate it using paprika.

3. Add the chopped onions into the baking dish and heat for about 2 minutes in the Cuisinart Air Fryer Oven.

4. Add the beef into the dish when the onions are transparent, and cook for 5 minutes.

5. Once the beef is starting to tender, pour in the sour cream and cook for another 7 minutes.

6. At this point, the liquid should have reduced. Season with salt and pepper and serve.

Nutrition:

Calories: 254

Fat: 21g

Protein:33g

Fiber:0g

11. Cheesy Ground Beef and Mac Taco Casserole

Preparation Time: 10 Minutes

Cooking Time: 25 Minutes

Servings: 5

Ingredients:

- 1-ounce shredded Cheddar cheese

- 1-ounce shredded Monterey Jack cheese

- 2 tablespoons chopped green onions

- 1/2 (10.75 ounce) can condensed tomato soup

- 1/2-pound lean ground beef

- 1/2 cup crushed tortilla chips

- 1/4-pound macaroni, cooked according to manufacturer's Directions:

- 1/4 cup chopped onion

- 1/4 cup sour cream (optional)

- 1/2 (1.25 ounce) package taco seasoning mix

• 1/2 (14.5 ounce) can diced tomatoes

Directions:

1. Lightly grease baking pan of air fryer with cooking spray. Add onion and ground beef. For 10 minutes, cook on 360°F. Halfway through cooking time, stir and crumble ground beef.

2. Add taco seasoning, diced tomatoes, and tomato soup. Mix well. Mix in pasta.

3. Sprinkle crushed tortilla chips. Sprinkle cheese.

4. Cook for 15 minutes at 390°F until tops are lightly browned and cheese is melted.

5. Serve and enjoy.

Nutrition:

Calories: 329

Fat: 17g

Protein: 15.6g

12. Beef Ribeye Steak

Preparation Time: 5 Minutes

Cooking Time: 20 Minutes

Servings: 4

Ingredients:

• 4 (8-ounce) ribeye steaks

• 1 tablespoon McCormick Grill Mates Montreal Steak Seasoning

• Salt

• Pepper

Directions:

1. Season the steaks with the steak seasoning and salt and pepper to taste. Place 2 steaks in the Cuisinart Air Fryer Oven. You can use an accessory grill pan, a layer rack, or the air fryer basket.

2. Cook for 4 minutes. Open the air fryer and flip the steaks.

3. Cook for an additional 4 to 5 minutes. Check for doneness to determine how much additional cook time is need. Remove the cooked

steaks from the Cuisinart Air Fryer Oven, then repeat for the remaining

2 steaks.

4. Cool before serving.

Nutrition:

Calories: 293

Fat: 22g

Protein:23g

Fiber:0g

13. Air Fryer Roast Beef

Preparation: 5 Minutes Cooking: 40 Minutes Servings: 6

Ingredients:

• Roast beef • 1 tbsp. olive oil • Seasonings of choice

Directions:

1. Ensure your Cuisinart Air Fryer Oven is preheated to 160 degrees.

2. Place roast in bowl and toss with olive oil and desired seasonings.

3. Put seasoned roast into air fryer.

4. Set temperature to 160°F, and set time to 30 minutes and cook 30 minutes.

5. Turn roast when the timer sounds and cook another 10 minutes.

Nutrition:

Calories: 267

Fat: 8g

Protein:21g Sugar:1g

14. Beef Korma

Preparation Time: 10 Minutes

Cooking Time: 20 Minutes

Servings: 6

Ingredients:

• ½ cup yogurt

• 1 tablespoon curry powder

• 1 tablespoon olive oil

• 1 onion, chopped

• 2 cloves garlic, minced

• 1 tomato, diced

• ½ cup frozen baby peas, thawed

Directions:

1. In a medium bowl, combine the steak, yogurt, and curry powder. Stir and set aside.

2. In a 6-inch metal bowl, combine the olive oil, onion, and garlic.

3. Cook for 3 to 4 minutes or until crisp and tender.

4. Add the steak along with the yogurt and the diced tomato. Cook for

12 to 13 minutes or until steak is almost tender.

5. Stir in the peas and cook for 2 to 3 minutes or until hot.

Nutrition:

Calories: 289

Fat: 11g

Protein:38g

Fiber:2g

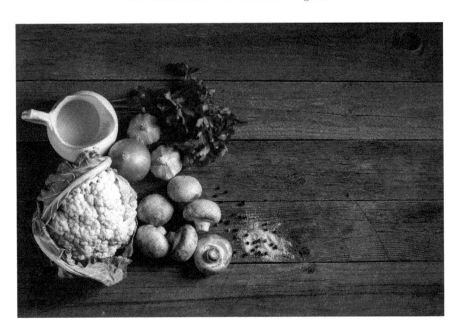

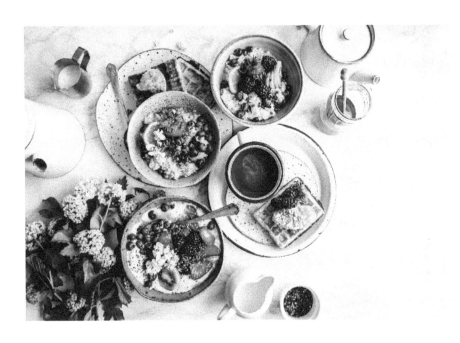

Poultry Recipes

15. Feta Chicken with Zucchini

Preparation Time: 20 Minutes

Cooking Time: 15 Minutes

Servings: 4

Ingredients

- 2 tbsp olive oil

- 1 lemon

- 4 boneless, skinless chicken breasts (about 1 1/2 pounds)

- ¼ tsp kosher salt

- 2 medium zucchinis

- ¼ cup fresh flat-leaf parsley leaves, chopped

- .13 tsp black pepper

- 1/3 cup (about 2 ounces) crumbled Feta

Directions

1.   Heat oven to 400° F. Drizzle ½ tbsp of the oil in a roasting pan. Remove the zest from the lemon in thin strips; set aside. Thinly slice the lemon. Place half the slices in the pan.

2.   Place the chicken on top of the lemon slices and season with 1/8 tsp of the salt.

3.   Slice each zucchini in half lengthwise, then slice each half into ¼-inch-thick half-moons. In a bowl, combine the zucchini, parsley, and pepper and the remaining oil, lemon slices, and salt; toss.

4.   Spread the mixture around the chicken and sprinkle the Feta over the top.

5.   Roast until the chicken is cooked through, 15 to 20 minutes. Transfer it to a cutting board and cut each piece into thirds.

6.   Divide the chicken, zucchini mixture, and lemons among individual plates and sprinkle with the zest.

Nutrition:

Calories: 270 kcal

Calories from fat: 27%

Fat: 8g

Saturated fat: 3g

Cholesterol: 110mg   Sodium: 378mg

Carbohydrates: 5g   Fiber: 2g Sugars: 3g

Protein: 42g

16. Cinnamon Chicken

Preparation Time: 10 Minutes

Cooking Time: 30 Minutes

Servings: 4

Ingredients

- 4 skinless, boneless chicken breast halves

- 1 tsp ground cinnamon

- 2 tbsp Italian-style seasoning

- 1 1/2 tsp garlic powder

- 3 tsp salt

- 1 tsp ground black pepper

Direction:

1. Preheat oven to 350 degrees F (175 degrees C).

2.   Place chicken in a lightly greased 9x13 inch baking dish. Sprinkle evenly with ground cinnamon, seasoning, garlic powder, salt and pepper. (Note: You can be liberal with the seasoning, garlic powder, salt and pepper; however, the cinnamon should only be a dusting and not clumped.)

3.   Bake at 350 degrees F (175 degrees C) for about 30 minutes or until chicken is cooked through and juices run clear.

Nutrition:

Calories: 143 kcal

Protein: 27.7g

Carbohydrates: 3g

Fat: 1.7g   Cholesterol: 68.4mg

Sodium: 1821.7mg

17. Chinese Five Spice Chicken

Preparation Time: 1 hour 15 Minutes

Cooking Time: 30 Minutes

Servings: 4-6

Ingredients

- 1 kg chicken piece

- 1 medium onion, finely chopped

- 1 -3 cloves of garlic, finely chopped

- 1/3 cup soy sauce

- 2 tbsp peanut oil

- 2 tsp five-spice powder

Direction:

1. Place the chicken pieces in a large dish or plastic bag.

2.   Mix the remaining ingredients and pour over the chicken.

3.   Marinate refrigerated overnight or for 1 to 2 hours if time is short.

4.   Transfer the chicken to a baking dish and brush with the marinade.

5.   Cook uncovered in a preheated 350F (180C) oven, brushing once or twice with the marinade until the chicken is done, about one hour.

Nutrition:

Calories: 331 kcal Protein: 38.24g Carbohydrates: 12.61g

Fat: 13.22g

Cholesterol: 112mg

Sodium: 787mg

18. Chicken with Acorn Squash and Tomatoes

Preparation: 20 Minutes Cooking: 10 Minutes Servings: 4

Ingredients

•   1 small acorn squash (about 1 1/2 pounds), halved, seeded, and

sliced 1/4 inch thick

•   1-pint grape tomatoes, halved

•   4 cloves of garlic, sliced •   3 tbsp olive oil

•   kosher salt and black pepper

•   4-6-ounce boneless, skinless chicken breasts

•   ½ tsp ground coriander

•   2 tbsp chopped fresh oregano

Direction:

1.   Heat oven to 425° F.

2.   On a large rimmed baking sheet, toss the squash, tomatoes and garlic with 2 tablespoons of the oil, ½ tsp salt and ¼ tsp pepper.

3.   Roast the vegetables until the squash is tender, 20 to 25 minutes.

4.   Meanwhile, heat the remaining tablespoon of oil in a large skillet over medium heat.

5.   Season the chicken with the coriander, ½ tsp salt and ¼ tsp pepper. Cook until golden brown and cooked through, 6 to 7 minutes per side.

6.   Serve the chicken with the squash and tomatoes and sprinkle with the oregano.

Nutrition:

Calories: 361 kcal   Fat: 15g   Saturated fat: 3g Cholesterol: 94mg

Sodium: 572mg Protein: 37g Carbohydrates: 22g Sugars: 6g

Fiber: 4g   Iron: 3mg Calcium: 96mg.

19. Chicken Cordon Bleu

Preparation Time: 10 Minutes

Cooking Time: 35 Minutes

Servings: 4

Ingredients

- 4 skinless, boneless chicken breast halves

- ¼ tsp salt

- 1/8 tsp ground black pepper

- 6 slices Swiss cheese

- 4 slices cooked ham

- ½ cup seasoned bread crumbs

Direction

1.   Preheat oven to 350 degrees F (175 degrees C). Coat a 7x11 inch baking dish with nonstick cooking spray.

2.   Pound chicken breasts to 1/4-inch thickness.

3.   Sprinkle each piece of chicken on both sides with salt and pepper. Place 1 cheese slice and 1 ham slice on top of each breast. Roll up each breast, and secure them with a toothpick. Place in a baking dish, and sprinkle chicken evenly with bread crumbs.

4.   Bake for 30 to 35 minutes, or until chicken is no longer pink. Remove from oven, and place 1/2 cheese slice on top of each breast. Return to oven for 3 to 5 minutes, or until cheese has melted. Remove toothpicks, and serve immediately.

Nutrition:

Calories: 195 kcal   Protein: 15.61g   Carbohydrates: 4.78g

Fat: 13.22g Cholesterol: 48mg Sodium: 490mg

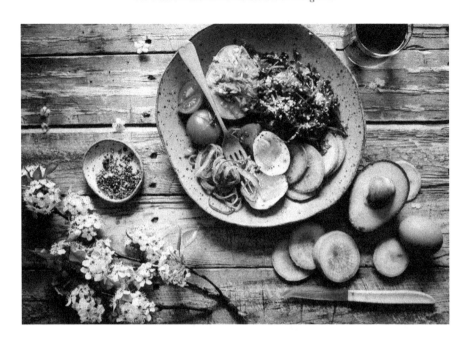

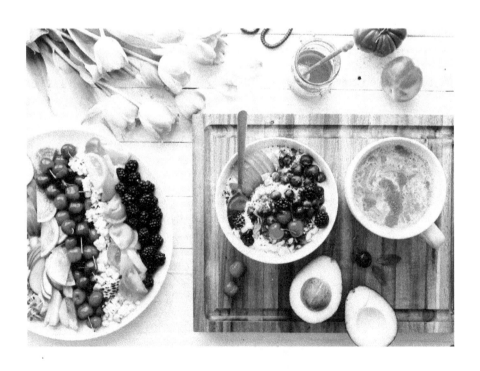

Fish and Seafood Recipes

20. Fish Bone Broth

Preparation time: 10 min Cooking time: 4 hrs.

Serving: 2

Ingredients:

• 2 pounds of the fish head or carcass

• Salt to taste • 7 – 8 quarts water + extra to blanch

• 2 inches ginger, sliced

• 2 tablespoons lemon juice

Direction:

1. To blanch the fish: Add water and fish heads into a large pot. Place

the pot over high heat.

2.Turn the heat off when it boils and discard the water.

3.Place the fish back in the pot. Pour 7-8 quarts of water.

4.Place the pot over high heat. Add ginger, salt, and lemon juice.

5.Reduce the heat as the mixture boils, and cover it with a lid.

6.Remove from heat. When it cools down, strain into a large jar with a wire mesh strainer.

7.Refrigerate for 5-6 days. Unused broth can be frozen.

Nutrition: Calories 254, Fat 4, Carbs 26, Protein 6, Sodium 455

21. Garlic Butter Shrimp

Preparation time: 10 min Cooking Time: 10 min

Serving: 2

Ingredients:

- 1 cup unsalted butter, divided

- Kosher salt to taste • ½ cup chicken stock

- Freshly ground pepper to taste

- ¼ cup chopped fresh parsley leaves

- 3 pounds medium shrimp, peeled, deveined garlic

- Juice of 2 lemons

Direction:

1.Add 4 tablespoons butter into a large skillet and place the skillet over

medium-high flame. Once butter melts, stir in salt, shrimp, and pepper and cook for 2 - 3 minutes. Stir every minute or so. Remove the shrimp with a spoon and place it on a tray.

2.Add garlic into the pot and cook until you get a nice aroma. Pour lemon juice and stock and stir.

3.Lower the heat and cook until the stock falls to half its initial volume until it comes to a boil.

4.Add the rest of the butter, a tablespoon each time, and stir until it melts each time.

5.Add shrimp and stir lightly until well coated.

6.Sprinkle parsley on top and serve.

Nutrition: Calories 484, Fat 21, Carbs 4, Protein 33, Sodium 370

22. Grilled Shrimp

Preparation time: 10 min

Cooking Time: 5 min

Serving: 2

Ingredients:

Shrimp Seasoning

- 2 teaspoons garlic powder

- 2 teaspoons Italian seasoning

- 2 teaspoons kosher salt

- ½ - 1 teaspoon cayenne pepper

Grilling

- 4 tablespoons extra-virgin olive oil

- 2 pounds shrimp, peeled, deveined

- 2 tablespoons fresh lemon juice

- Oil to grease the grill grated

Direction:

1. You can grill the shrimp in a grill or boil it in an oven. Choose whatever method suits you and preheat the grill or oven to high heat.

2. In case you are broiling it in an oven, prepare a baking sheet by lining it with foil and greasing the foil as well, with some fat.

3. Add garlic powder, cayenne pepper, salt, and Italian seasoning into a large bowl and mix well.

4. Add lemon juice and oil and mix well.

5. Stir in the shrimp. Make sure that the shrimp are well coated with the mixture.

6. If using the grill, fix the shrimp on skewers; else, place them on the baking sheet.

7.Grease the grill grates with some oil. Grill the shrimp or broil them in an oven until they turn pink. It should take 180 seconds for each side.

Nutrition: Calories 309, Fat 12, Carbs 8, Protein 16, Sodium 340

23. Garlic Ghee Pan-Fried Cod

Preparation time: 5 min

Cooking Time: 10 min

Serving: 2

Ingredients:

- 2 cod fillets (4.8 ounces each)

- 3 cloves garlic, peeled, minced

- Salt to taste

- 1 ½ tablespoons ghee

- ½ tablespoon garlic powder (optional)

Direction:

1.Place a pan over medium-high flame. Add ghee.

2.Once ghee melts, stir in half the garlic and cook for about 6 – 10 seconds.

3.Add fillets and season with garlic powder and salt.

4.Soon the color of the fish will turn white. This color should be visible for about half the height of the fish.

5.Turn the fish over and cook, adding remaining garlic.

6.When the entire fillet turns white, remove it from the pan.

Nutrition: Calories 193, Fat 16, Carbs 6, Protein 21, Sodium 521

24. Mussel and Potato Stew

Preparation time: 10 min

Cooking Time: 20 min

Serving: 2

Ingredients:

- potatoes

- broccoli

- olive oil

- filets

- garlic

Direction:

1.Submerge potatoes in cold water in a medium saucepan. Put the salt, and boil. Allow cooling for 15 minutes till soft. Let drain.

2.Boil a saucepan of salted water. Put broccoli rabe, and allow to cook till just soft; it should turn bright green. Drain thoroughly, and slice into 2-inch lengths.

3.In a big, deep skillet, mix garlic, anchovies, and oil. Let cook over high heat for approximately a minute, crushing anchovies. In a skillet, scatter the mussels, put chopped parsley, broccoli rabe, and potatoes on top. Put half cup water, and add salt to season. Place the cover, and allow to cook till mussels are open.

Nutrition:

Calories 254, Fat 9, Carbs 12, Protein 11, Sodium 326

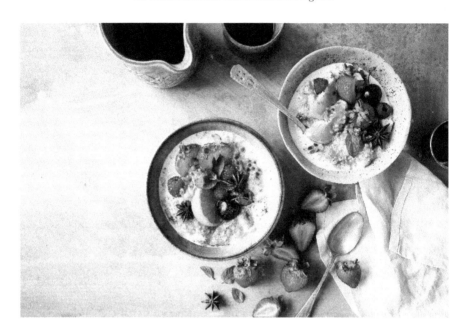

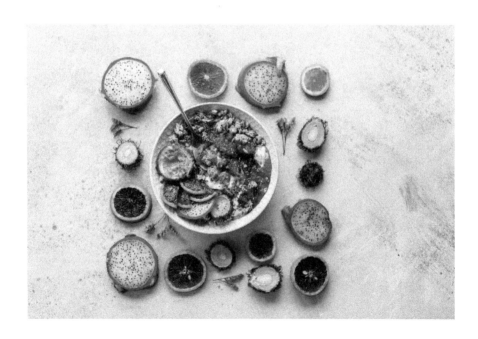

Side Dish Recipes

25. Popcorn Mushrooms

Preparation time: 10 minutes

Cooking time: 10 minutes

Servings: 4

Ingredients:

- 16 oz. of mushrooms

- 2 tablespoons of almond flour

- 2 tablespoons of water

- ½ teaspoon of minced garlic

- 1 tablespoon of olive oil

- ¼ teaspoon of chili flakes

Directions:

1. Mix together the almond flour, water, minced garlic, and chili flakes in a bowl.

2. Stir the mixture.

3. Coat the mushrooms with the almond flour mixture.

4. Spray the olive oil inside the air fryer basket.

5. Put the mushrooms and cook them for 10 minutes at 365oF.

6. Stir the mushrooms every 2 minutes.

7. Serve the cooked popcorn mushrooms only hot!

Nutrition:

Calories: 135 Fat: 10.8 g Fiber: 2.6 g Carbs: 6.9 g

Protein: 6.6 g

26. Thyme Mushrooms and Carrot Bowl

Preparation time: 10 minutes

Cooking time: 20 minutes

Servings: 4

Ingredients:

- 1 cup of baby carrot oz. of mushrooms; sliced

- 1 teaspoon of thyme

- 1 teaspoon of salt

- 1 cup of chicken stock

- 1 teaspoon of chili flakes

- 1 teaspoon of coconut oil

Directions:

1   Place the baby carrot in the air fryer basket.

2   Add thyme, salt, and chili flakes.

3   Cook the baby carrot for 10 minutes at 380oF.

4   Then add the sliced mushrooms and coconut oil.

5   Stir it well and cook the vegetables for 10 minutes more at 370oF.

6   Stir the vegetables after 5 minutes of cooking.

Chill the cooked entremots and enjoy!

Nutrition:

Calories: 25 g

Fat: 1.5 g

Fiber: 0.7 g

Carbs: 2.2 g rProtein: 2 g

Soup and Salad Recipes

27. Normandy Salad

Preparation Time: 25 minutes Cooking Time: 5 minutes

Servings: 4 to 6

Level of difficulty: Normal

Category: Green

Ingredients:

For the walnuts:

* 2 tablespoons butter

* ¼ cup sugar or honey

* 1 cup walnut pieces

* ½ teaspoon kosher salt

For the dressing:

- 3 tablespoons extra-virgin olive oil

- 1½ tablespoons champagne vinegar

- 1½ tablespoons Dijon mustard

- ¼ teaspoon kosher salt

For the salad:

- 1 head red leaf lettuce, shredded into pieces

- 3 heads endive, ends trimmed and leaves separated

- 2 apples, cored and divided into thin wedges

- 1 (8-ounce) Camembert wheel, cut into thin wedges

Directions:

1. For the walnuts, dissolve the butter in a skillet over medium-high heat. Stir in the sugar and cook until it dissolves.

2.   Add the walnuts and cook for about 5 minutes, stirring, until toasty. Season with salt and transfer to a plate to cool.

3.   For the dressing, whip the oil, vinegar, mustard, and salt in a large bowl until combined.

4.   For the salad, add the lettuce and endive to the bowl with the dressing, and toss to coat. Transfer to a serving platter.

5.   Decoratively arrange the apple and Camembert wedges over the lettuce and scatter the walnuts on top. Serve immediately.

Nutrition:

Calories: 699 Fat: 52 g

Carbs: 44 g

Protein: 23 g

28. Coleslaw Worth A Second Helping

Preparation Time: 20 minutes

Cooking Time: 10 minutes

Servings: 6

Level of difficulty: Easy

Category: Green

Ingredients:

- 5 cups shredded cabbage

- 2 carrots, shredded

- ½ cup mayonnaise

- ½ cup sour cream

- 3 tablespoons apple cider vinegar

- 1 teaspoon kosher salt

- ½ teaspoon celery seed

Directions:

1.   Add together the cabbage, carrots, and parsley in a large bowl. Whisk together the mayonnaise, sour cream, vinegar, salt, and celery in a small bowl until smooth.

2.   Pour sauce over veggies until covered. Transfer to a serving bowl and bake until ready to serve.

Nutrition:

Calories: 192

Fat: 18 g

Carbs: 7 g

Protein: 2 g

29. Romaine Lettuce and Radicchios Mix

Preparation Time: 6 minutes

Cooking Time: 0 minutes

Servings: 4

Level of difficulty: Easy

Category: Green

Ingredients:

- 2 tablespoons olive oil

- A pinch of salt and black pepper

- 2 spring onions, chopped

- 3 tablespoons Dijon mustard

- Juice of 1 lime

- ½ cup basil, chopped

- 4 cups romaine lettuce heads, chopped

- 3 radicchios, sliced

Directions:

1.   In a salad bowl, blend the lettuce with the spring onions and the other ingredients. Toss and serve.

Nutrition:

Calories: 87

Fats: 2 g

Carbs: 1 g

Protein: 2 g

30. Asparagus and Smoked Salmon Salad

Preparation: 15 minutes Cooking: 10 minutes Servings: 8

Level of difficulty: Normal

Category: Lean

Ingredients:

- 1 lb. fresh asparagus, shaped and cut into 1-inch pieces

- 1/2 cup pecans, smashed into pieces

- 2 heads red leaf lettuce, washed and split

- 1/2 cup frozen green peas, thawed

- 1/4 lb. smoked salmon, cut into 1-inch chunks

- 1/4 cup olive oil

- 2 tablespoons lemon juice

- 1 teaspoon Dijon mustard

- 1/2 teaspoon salt

- 1/4 teaspoon pepper

Directions:

1. Boil a pot of water. Stir in asparagus and cook for 5 minutes until tender. Let it drain and set aside.

2. In a skillet, cook the pecans over medium heat for 5 minutes, continually stirring until lightly toasted.

3. Combine the asparagus, toasted pecans, salmon, peas, and red leaf lettuce and toss in a large bowl.

4. In another bowl, combine lemon juice, pepper, Dijon mustard, salt, and olive oil. You can coat the salad with the dressing, then serve.

Nutrition:

Calories: 159 Carbs: 7 g Fat: 12.9 g Protein: 6 g

31. Shrimp Cobb Salad

Preparation Time: 25 minutes

Cooking Time: 10 minutes

Servings: 2

Level of difficulty: Normal

Category: Leanest

Ingredients:

- 4 slices center-cut bacon

- 1 lb. large shrimp, peeled and deveined

- 1/2 teaspoon ground paprika

- 1/4 teaspoon ground black pepper

- 1/4 teaspoon salt, divided

- 2 1/2 tablespoons fresh lemon juice

- 1 1/2 tablespoons extra-virgin olive oil

- 1/2 teaspoon whole-grain Dijon mustard

- 1 (10 oz.) package romaine lettuce hearts, chopped

- 2 cups cherry tomatoes, quartered

- 1 ripe avocado, cut into wedges

- 1 cup shredded carrots

Directions:

1.   Cook the bacon for 4 minutes on each side in a large skillet over medium heat till crispy.

2.   Take away from the skillet and place on paper towels; let cool for 5 minutes. Break the bacon into bits. Throw out most of the bacon fat, leaving behind only 1 tablespoon in the skillet.

3.   Bring the skillet back to medium-high heat. Add black pepper and paprika to the shrimp for seasoning.

4. Cook the shrimp for around 2 minutes on each side until it is opaque. Sprinkle with 1/8 teaspoon of salt for seasoning.

5. Combine the remaining 1/8 teaspoon of salt, mustard, olive oil, and lemon juice in a small bowl. Stir in the romaine hearts.

6. On each serving plate, place 1 and 1/2 cups of romaine lettuce. Add on top the same amounts of avocado, carrots, tomatoes, shrimp, and bacon.

Nutrition:

Calories: 528

Carbohydrate: 22.7 g

Fat: 28.7 g

Protein: 48.9 g

Lean and Green Recipe

32. Green Mango Smoothie Bowl

Preparation: 5 minutes Cooking: 5 minutes Serving: 1

Ingredients

- 1.5 mango bowls frozen. • 1 cup of spinach packed loosely

- 1 cup dummy wrapped up • 2 tbsp or chia seeds 2 tbsp

- 1 tbsp citrus fruit juice

- 1 cup of milk with no air (almond or coconut)

- Obstacles (optional)

- Mango in slices

- Floats of coconut

- Beers Beers

- Seeds or noodles

- Granola: Granola

Direction:

1. In a high-speed blender, add all ingredients. Mix until creamy and smooth.

2. Smoothie in a bowl transferred.

3. Top bowls of smoothie with some toppings. Good luck!

Nutrition

Serving Size: 1 smoothie bowl

Calories: 358 Sugar: 38g Fat: 13g

Saturated Fat: 1g Carbohydrates: 50g

Fiber: 8g Protein: 13g

33. Whole Grain Toast with Avocado Slices

Preparation Time: 5 minutes

Cooking Time: 5 minutes

Servings: 4

Ingredients

- 4 bread in slices, all wheat

- Two Middle Ages

- 1 lime medium

- Salt 1/8 cucharcino

- 1/8 tea cubicle black pepper.

Direction:

1. Toast bread. Toast bread.

2. Place avocados in pieces and put on toast.

3. Season with salt and pepper to taste. Spritz with lime juice.

Nutrition

Calories: 247kcal

Carbohydrates: 24g

Protein: 6g

Fat: 16g

Saturated Fat: 3g

Sodium: 227mg

Fiber: 9g

Sugar: 3g

34. Cinnamon and Walnut Porridge

Preparation Time: 5 mins

Cooking Time: 5 mins

Serving: 4 cups

Ingredients

- 2 cups of oats rolling •Mandy milk 2 cups

- Water for 2 cups

- 1/4 tea cuchar.

- Vanilla extract from 1/2 teaspoon.

- Cinnamon 1/2 teaspoon ground •   Walnuts 1/2 cup

Direction:

1. In a medium bowl, add all ingredients (except for the cinnamon

   and walnuts). Heat over medium heat and stir well.

2. Apply a blend to a fry.

3. Stirring sometimes, soak for 5 minutes.

4. Serve with a walnut spoon and sprinkle on top with cinnamon.

    Alternatively, you will add cinnamon to your porridge mixture

    at the start if you do not want cinnamon to show up as a garnish.

Nutrition

Calories: 324kcal

Carbohydrates: 40.29g

Protein: 15.05g

Fat: 20.34g

Sodium: 57mg Fiber: 8.9g

Sugar: 7.45g

Vegetables and Sides Recipes

35. Zucchini Boat

Preparation Time: 25 Minutes

Cooking Time: 20 Minutes

Servings: 2

Ingredients:

2 medium zucchinis

2 tablespoons of olive oil

1/2 medium onion, diced

2 garlic cloves, minced

1 can corn, drained

1 cup enchilada sauce

1/2 tsp. salt or to taste

1 /2 cup white mushrooms

½ cup bok Choy, chopped

1 teaspoon cumin

1/2 cup parmesan cheese

Directions:

1.   Wash and cut the zucchini lengthwise.

2.   heat oil in a skillet and sauté onions.

3.   Then add garlic cloves and cook until aroma comes

4.   add in vegetables and cook until tender.

5.   then add salt and enchilada sauce and cumin

6.   mix well

7.   turn off heat and let it get cool

8.   Scoop out the seeds of zucchinis.

9.   Fill the cavity of zucchinis with bowl mixture.

10.   Top it with a handful of Parmesan cheese.

11.   Arrange 4 zucchinis in the air fryer basket.

12.   Select the AIR FRY for 20 minutes and adjust the temperature

to 390 degrees F.

13.   Once done, serve and enjoy.

Serving Suggestion: Serve it with ketchup

Variation Tip: None

Nutritional Information Per Serving:

Calories 472 Fat 28 2g Sodium 1157mg Carbs 40.5g

Fiber 10.5g Sugar 7.7g Protein 26.5g

36. Air Fryer Stuffed Peppers

Preparation Time: 20 Minutes

Cooking Time: 18 Minutes

Servings: 6

Ingredients:

6 Green Bell Peppers 1 tablespoon olive oil

1/3 cup green onion diced ¼ cup fresh parsley

¼ teaspoon ground sage ¼ teaspoon garlic salt

1 cup marinara sauce 1/2 cup shredded mozzarella Cheese

Directions:

1.   Take a skillet and add oil in it

2.   Then add green onion, parsley, sage, and salt.

3.   Let it cook for 2 minutes then add marinara, mix well.

4.   Cut the top off of bell peppers and clean the cavity,

5.   Scoop the skillet mixture into each of the peppers and top with
cheese

6.   Place it in the basket of the air fryer.

7.   Cook for 18 minutes at 355 degrees F.

8.   Once done, serve.

Serving Suggestion: Serve it with chicken wings

Variation Tip: use sesame oil with olive oil

Nutritional Information Per Serving:

Calories 102 Fat 4.2g Sodium 186mg Carbs 15.1g

Fiber 2.8g Sugar 9.7g

Protein 2.7g

37. Air Fryer Spaghetti Squash

Preparation: 25 Minutes Cooking: 25 Minutes Servings: 6

Ingredients:

1 (3 pounds) spaghetti squash

1 teaspoon olive oil ¼ teaspoon sea salt

1/8 Teaspoon ground black pepper

1/8 Teaspoon smoked paprika

Directions:

1.   Create a dotted line lengthwise around the squash with knife.

2.   Cook the squash in the microwave at high for 5 minutes.

3.   Transfer it to a cutting board

4.   Cut the squash in half lengthwise,

5.   Spoon pulp and seeds out of the one half and discard.

6.   Brush it with olive oil

7.   Season it with salt, pepper, and paprika.

8.   Preheat the air fryer to 360 degrees F

9.   Once preheated put the squash half skin side-down in the basket.

10.   Cook for 20 minutes.

11.   Serve and enjoy.

Serving Suggestion: Serve it with sour cream

Variation Tip: Use oil spray instead of olive oil

Nutritional Information Per Serving:

Calories 77 Fat 2.1g Sodium 117mg Carbs 15.7g

Fiber 0g Sugar 0g Protein 1.5g

38. Vegan Meatballs

Preparation Time: 20 minutes.

Cooking Time: 48 minutes.

Serves: 4

Ingredients:

- 1 cup cooked quinoa

- 1 (15-ounce) can black beans

- 2 tablespoons water

- 3 garlic cloves, minced

- 1/2 cup shallot, diced

- 1/4 teaspoon salt

- 2 1/2 teaspoon fresh oregano

- 1/2 teaspoon red pepper flake

- 1/2 teaspoon fennel seeds

- 1/2 cup vegan parmesan cheese, shredded

- 2 tablespoons tomato paste

- 3 tablespoons fresh basil, chopped

- 2 tablespoons worcestershire sauce

Direction:

1.   At 350 degrees F, preheat your oven.

2.   Spread the beans in a baking sheet and bake for 15 minutes.

3.   Meanwhile, sauté garlic, shallots and water to a skillet for 3 minutes.

4.   Transfer to the food processor along with fennel, red pepper flakes, baked beans, oregano and salt.

5.   Blend these ingredients just until incorporated.

6.   Stir in quinoa, and rest of the ingredients then mix evenly.

7.   Make golf-ball sized meatballs out of this mixture.

8.   Spread these meatballs in a grease baking sheet and bake for 20-30 minutes until brown.

9.   Flip the meatballs once cooked half way through.

10.   Serve warm.

Serving Suggestion: Serve the meatballs with pita bread and chili sauce.

Variation Tip: Add chopped mushrooms to the batter as well.

Nutritional Information Per Serving:

Calories 338

Fat 24g Sodium 620mg Carbs 58.3g

Fiber 2.4g Sugar 1.2g Protein 5.4g

39. Tofu Fried Rice

Preparation Time: 10 minutes.

Cooking Time: 13 minutes.

Serves: 4

Ingredients:

*   1 package baked tofu

*   4 cup cauliflower rice

*   1 cup frozen peas

*   1 cup carrots, shredded

*   1 teaspoon onion powder

*   1 teaspoon garlic powder

*   1/2 cup soy sauce

*   1/4 cup scallions, chopped

- Salt and black pepper to taste

Direction:

1.   Sauce tofu with peas, carrots, garlic powder, soy sauce, scallions, black pepper and salt in a cooking pan for 10 minutes.

2.   Stir in cauliflower rice and mix well.

3.   Cover and cook for 3 minutes on medium heat.

4.   Serve warm.

Serving Suggestion: Serve the rice with kale salad.

Variation Tip: Add boiled couscous to the mixture.

Nutritional Information Per Serving:

Calories 378 Fat 3.8g Sodium 620mg

Carbs 13.3g Fiber 2.4g Sugar 1.2g Protein 5.4g

40. Rice and Beans

Preparation: 15 minutes. Cooking: 22 minutes.Serves: 4

Ingredients:

* 1 cup dry brown rice •1 ½ cup water

* 1 can of black beans • 1 teaspoon paprika

* 1 teaspoon garlic powder

* 1 teaspoon oregano • 1 teaspoon cumin

* 1 teaspoon onion powder

Direction:

1. At 350 degrees F, preheat your oven.

2. Add water and rice to the Instant Pot's insert.

3. Set a trivet over the rice and place a baking dish on top.

4. Add beans and rest of the ingredients to this bowl.

5. Cover and seal the lid and cook for 22 minutes at Low pressure.

6. Once done, release all the pressure and remove the lid.

7. Mix the beans and transfer to a serving plate.

8. Serve the beans with the rice.

9. Enjoy.

Serving Suggestion: Serve the beans with the spinach salad.

Variation Tip: Add crispy fried onion on top for better taste.

Nutritional Information Per Serving:

Calories 304

Fat 31g Sodium 834mg Carbs 21.4g Fiber 0.2g

Sugar 0.3g Protein 4.6g

Snacks and Dessert Recipes

41. Peanut Butter

Preparation: 5 minutes Cooking: 0 minutes Serving: 14

Ingredients:

- cups raw or roasted peanuts 1 teaspoon vanilla

- sea salt to preference

Directions:

1. Add all ingredients to a high-speed food processor and blend until smooth. This may take several minutes, and you may need to scrape the sides of the blender frequently.

Nutritional Information Per Serving:

178 Calories, 15 grams of fat, 5 grams of Carbs, 8 grams of Protein

42. Vegan Crackers

Preparation time: 15 minutes

Cooking time 10 minutes

Serving Size: 30 servings

Ingredients:

- 1 cup quinoa flour ½ cup sorghum flour

- ½ cup nutritional yeast ½ teaspoon Himalayan salt

- ½ cup kale, finely chopped

- 2 tablespoon olive oil

- 2/3 cup cold water

Directions:

1.   Preheat the oven to 450 Fahrenheit or 232 Celsius. Line a baking

sheet with parchment paper.

2.   Toast quinoa on the stove and stir frequently.

3.   Allow the flour to cool for 5 minutes before adding to a food processor.

4.   Add sorghum flour, nutritional yeast, and salt. Pulse a few times.

5.   Add kale and pulse.

6.   Add in oil and water until the dough starts to come together.

7.   Remove the dough and form it into a ball. Let the dough rest for a few minutes.

8.   Separate the dough into four pieces. Knead each piece with your hands.

9.   Roll each part as thin as possible.

10.   Transfer the dough onto the baking sheets after rolling.

11.   Bake the crackers for 5 minutes on each side.

12.   Turn the oven off but allow the crackers to stay in the oven for one or two hours to get crispy.

13.   Remove from oven and allow cooking before breaking them into pieces.

Nutritional Information Per Serving (2 Scoops):

50 Calories, 2 grams of fat, 4 grams of Carbs, 2 grams of Protein

43. Spelt Banana Bread

Preparation Time: 10 minutes Cooking Time: 45 minutes

Servings: 9

Ingredients:

- 1 ½ cups spelt flour

- 3 medium burro bananas, peeled

- ¾ cup pecans • 1 ½ teaspoons baking soda

- ½ cup maple syrup

- 1 teaspoon vanilla extract, unsweetened

- ¼ teaspoon salt • 3 tablespoons canola oil

Directions:

1. Preheat the oven to 350°F. Grease a 9-by-5-inch loaf pan with oil and then set aside.

2.   Take a large bowl, place the peeled bananas in it, mash them well using a fork, and then mix in vanilla, maple syrup, and oil until combined.

3.   Take a separate large bowl, place flour in it, add pecans, baking soda, and salt, and then stir until mixed.

4.   Pour in banana mixture, blend by using an electric mixer until incorporated and smooth, and then pour it into the prepared pan.

5.   Bake the bread for 40–45 minutes. When done, let it cool within 10 minutes. Cut the bread into nine slices and then serve.

Nutrition:

Calories: 185.9| Carbs: 22 g| Fat: 11.3 g| Protein: 1.3 g

44. Yeast-Free Spelt Bread

Preparation Time: 10 minutes

Cooking Time: 1 hour and 10 minutes

Servings: 12

Ingredients:

- ¾ cup rolled oats; quick-cooking, divided

- 3½ cups whole-spelt flour

- 1 teaspoon of sea salt

- 2 tablespoons baking powder

- ¼ cup sesame seeds

- 2 tablespoons maple syrup

- 2 tablespoons coconut oil, melted

- 2 cups almond milk; unsweetened, warmed

Directions:

1.   Preheat the oven to 350 F.

2.   Take a 9-by-5-inch-loaf pan, grease it with oil, and then set aside until needed.

3.   Take a large bowl, place flour in it, add baking powder, sesame seeds, ½ cup oats, salt, and then stir until mixed.

4.   Take a separate large bowl, pour in the milk, and then whisk in oil and honey until well combined.

5.   Beat in flour mixture, ½ cup at a time, by using an electric mixer until incorporated. Put your batter into the prepared loaf pan, and then spread remaining oats on top, pressing them into the batter.

6.   Bake the bread for 1 hour and 10 minutes until the top has turned golden-brown; check the bread's doneness by inserting a knife into its center, which should come out clean.

7.   Let the bread cool in the pan within 10 minutes, lift it out, and

cool the bread entirely on a wire rack.

8.   Cut the bread into twelve slices and then serve.

Nutrition:

Calories: 125| Carbs: 23 g| Fat: 5 g| Protein: 6 g

45. Flatbread

Preparation: 10 minutes Cooking: 72 minutes Servings: 6

Ingredients:

- 2 cups spelt-flour

- 2 teaspoons onion powder

- 1 tablespoon of sea salt

- 2 teaspoons dried oregano

- ¼ teaspoons cayenne pepper

- 2 teaspoons dried basil • 2 tablespoons grapeseed oil

- ¾ cup spring water

Directions:

1.   Take a large bowl, place flour in it, add all the seasoning in it, and then stir until well mixed.

2.   Add oil and then slowly mix in water until a dough ball forms.

3.   Transfer the dough onto a working space dusted with flour and then knead it for 5 minutes until elastic.

4.   Split the dough into six portions, roll each piece into a ball, and then roll each ball using a rolling pin into a 4-inch round.

5.   Take a medium skillet pan, place it over medium-high heat and when hot, place a flatbread round in it and then cook for 3 minutes per side until golden-brown and cooked.

6.   Transfer cooked flatbread to a plate and then cook the remaining pieces of bread in the same manner. Serve straight away.

Nutrition:

Calories: 110 | Carbs: 18 g | Fat: 3 g | Protein: 1 g

46. Vanilla Frappe

Nutrition:

Calories: 155

Fat: 4.4g

Carbohydrates: 15.2g

Protein: 15g

Preparation time: 5 minutes

Cooking time: 0 minutes

Servings: 1

Level of difficulty: Easy

Ingredients:

- 1 sachet Optavia Essential Vanilla Shake

- 8 ounces unsweetened almond milk

- ½ cup ice

- 1 tablespoon whipped topping

Directions: In a blender, add the Vanilla Shake sachet, almond milk, and ice and pulse until smooth. Transfer the mixture into a glass and top with whipped topping. Serve immediately.

47. Ginger Cheesecake

Preparation Time: 20 minutes

Cooking Time: 20 Minutes

Servings: 6

Ingredients:

• 2 tbsp. butter

• ½ cup ginger cookies

• 16 oz. cream cheese

• 2 eggs

• ½ cup sugar

• 1 tbsp. rum

• ½ tbsp. vanilla extract

• ½ tbsp. nutmeg

Directions:

1.Spread pan with the butter and sprinkle cookie crumbs on the bottom.

2.Whisk cream cheese with rum, vanilla, nutmeg and eggs, beat properly and sprinkle the cookie crumbs.

3.Put in air fryer and cook at 340° F for 20 minutes.

4.Allow cheese cake to cool in fridge for 2 hours before slicing.

5.Serve.

Nutrition:

Calories: 312

Total Fat: 9.8g

Total carbs: 18g

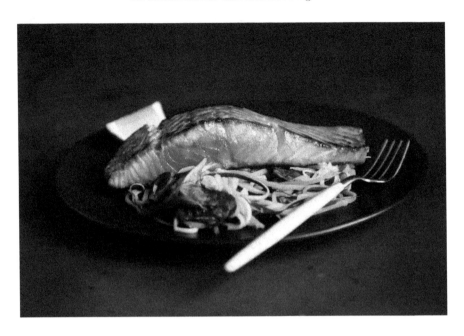

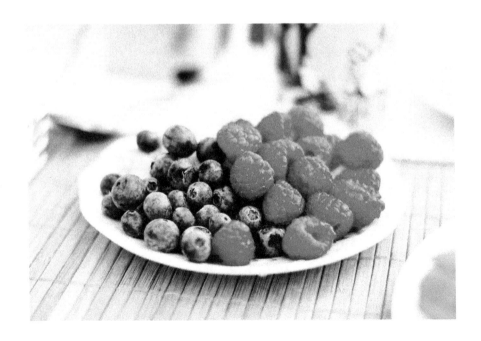

Fueling Recipes

48. Green Apple Smoothie

Preparation Time: 5 minutes.

Cooking Time: 0 minutes.

Serves: 2

Ingredients:

- 2 ripe bananas

- 1 ripe pear, peeled, chopped

- 2 cups kale leaves, chopped

- ½ cup of orange juice

- ½ cup of cold water

- 12 ice cubes

- 1 tablespoon ground flaxseed

Direction:

1. Blend bananas with pear, kale leaves, orange juice, cold water, ice cubes and flaxseed in a blender.

2. Serve.

Serving Suggestion: Serve this smoothie with morning muffins.

Variation Tip: Add some strawberries to the smoothie.

Nutritional Information Per Serving:

Calories 213 | Fat 2.5g |Sodium 15.6mg | Carbs 49.5g | Fiber 7.6g | Sugar 28g | Protein 3.5g

49. Spinach Smoothie

Preparation Time: 5 minutes.

Cooking Time: 0 minutes.

Serves: 2

Ingredients:

- 1 cup fresh spinach

- 1 banana

- ½ green apple

- 4 hulled strawberries

- 4 (1 inch) pieces frozen mango

- 1/3 cup whole milk

- 1 scoop vanilla protein powder

- 1 teaspoon honey

Direction:

1.   Blend spinach with banana with the green apple with strawberries, mango, milk, protein powder and honey in a blender.

2.   Serve.

Serving Suggestion: Enjoy this smoothie with breakfast muffins.

Variation Tip: Add some blueberries to the smoothie.

Nutritional Information Per Serving:

Calories 312 | Fat 25g | Sodium 132mg | Carbs 44g | Fiber 3.9g | Sugar 3g | Protein 18.9g

50. Kale and Cheese Muffins

Preparation Time: 10 minutes.

Cooking Time: 25 minutes.

Serves: 9

Ingredients:

- 9 large eggs

- 1 cup liquid egg whites

- 3/4 cup plain Greek yogurt

- 2 ounces goat cheese crumbled

- 1/2 teaspoon salt

- 10 ounces kale

- 2 cups cherry tomatoes

- cooking spray

Direction:

1.   At 375 degrees F, preheat your oven.

2.   Beat eggs with goat cheese, yogurt, and egg whites in a bowl.

3.   Stir in cherry tomatoes and kale, then divide this mixture into a muffin tray.

4.   Bake the muffin cups for 25 minutes in the preheated oven.

5.   Enjoy.

Serving Suggestion: Serve these muffins with a green smoothie.

Variation Tip: Add chopped nuts to the batter.

Nutritional Information Per Serving:

Calories 290 | Fat 15g |Sodium 595mg | Carbs 11g | Fiber 3g | Sugar 12g | Protein 29g

Conclusion

It is the last article in my series on Lean and Green Recipes. Thank you so much for sticking with me all this way, and I hope you found it helpful. I have compiled a series of useful resources at the end of this article, including some wonderful books, websites and podcasts. I can recommend readers who have more knowledge about sustainable living or cooking to interested readers. They helped me a lot over the last few years and I hope they can do the same for you too.

Lean cooking is a style of cooking that emphasizes relatively low-fat content and minimal use of oil. Lean meat, fish, vegetables and grains are cooked in the minimum amount of fat necessary to preserve them. It's not a very customizable way to cook because you can't change the fat content or oil used (you can however swap out all the lean ingredients with higher fat ones).

Green cooking is a style of cooking that emphasizes lessening the environmental impact of your meal preparation by focusing on local, seasonal produce, along with avoiding the use of processed foods or meats that have been produced overseas. As with Lean cooking, it's not very customizable since you're required to buy local and seasonal produce.

The basic idea behind Lean and Green cooking is to approach your weekly meal planning from a perspective of total calories instead of from a perspective of how many calories you are getting from fat or protein. You can use the concepts and recipes I provide to make your own lean meats and green foods, or you can improvise new things.

Because Lean and Green cooking approaches your weekly meal planning from a perspective of total calories instead of from a perspective of how many calories you are getting from fat or protein, it helps you develop a more mindful relationship with food. It's easier to overeat and to consume more calories than you need when you don't pay attention to the actual numbers of food that you're eating. Lean and Green cooking helps break this cycle and make you more aware of your relationship with food in a positive way.

It's also a very simple way to eat, once you figure out what combination of foods works best for your body. And this is where I've found the most appeal for myself personally. My body feels great when I eat a nutritious diet, but I'm also very aware of how many calories I'm eating, and simultaneously, how much fat or protein is in those calories. And if my stomach feels like it's about to boom (which it does sometimes!), I know that there's enough food in my meal that makes me satisfied and not too full.

I hope you can take some of my lessons into your own kitchen. And if you substitute a few ingredients or otherwise make adjustments to suit your tastes, feel free! After all, that's really what creating food is all about: using whatever ingredients you have for what dish you want to create. What matters is the love and care that go into it.

CPSIA information can be obtained
at www.ICGtesting.com
Printed in the USA
BVHW090947030621
608731BV00010B/1773

9 781801 892438